TEEN GUIDE:
SOCIAL ANXIETY

by Mary Gerard

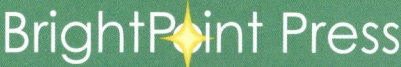

San Diego, CA

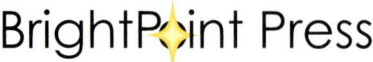

© 2026 BrightPoint Press
an imprint of ReferencePoint Press, Inc.
Printed in the United States

For more information, contact:
BrightPoint Press
PO Box 27779
San Diego, CA 92198
www.BrightPointPress.com

ALL RIGHTS RESERVED.

No part of this work covered by the copyright hereon may be reproduced or used in any form or by any means—graphic, electronic, or mechanical, including photocopying, recording, taping, web distribution, or information storage retrieval systems—without the written permission of the publisher.

Content Consultant: Matthew Carper, PhD, Assistant Professor in the Clinical Psychology Department, William James College

LIBRARY OF CONGRESS CATALOGING-IN-PUBLICATION DATA

Library of Congress Cataloging-in-Publication Data
Name: Gerard, Mary, author.
Title: Teen guide: social anxiety / by Mary Gerard.
Description: San Diego, CA: BrightPoint Press, 2026 | Series: Teen guide to mental health | Audience: Grade 7 to 9 | Includes bibliographical references and index.
Identifiers: ISBN: 9781678211486 (hardcover) | ISBN: 9781678211493 (eBook)
The complete Library of Congress record is available at www.loc.gov.

CONTENTS

CONTENT WARNING: THIS BOOK DESCRIBES SUICIDE AND SUICIDAL THOUGHTS, WHICH MAY BE TRIGGERING TO SOME READERS.

AT A GLANCE   4

INTRODUCTION   6
GRIDIRON STAR GRAPPLES WITH SOCIAL ANXIETY

CHAPTER ONE   12
WHAT IS SOCIAL ANXIETY?

CHAPTER TWO   26
EFFECTS OF SOCIAL ANXIETY

CHAPTER THREE   40
FINDING SUPPORT FOR SOCIAL ANXIETY

Glossary   58
Source Notes   59
For Further Research   60
Index   62
Image Credits   63
About the Author   64

AT A GLANCE

- Social anxiety disorder (SAD) is a mental health condition that causes distress in social situations. People with SAD are more than merely shy.

- Many symptoms may affect people with SAD. These include stress-related symptoms such as a raised heart rate in social situations.

- SAD is likely caused by a combination of genetic and environmental factors.

- More than 75 percent of people with SAD first developed symptoms as a child or a teen.

- SAD can isolate a teen from friends and family. It can also affect a teen's performance at school.

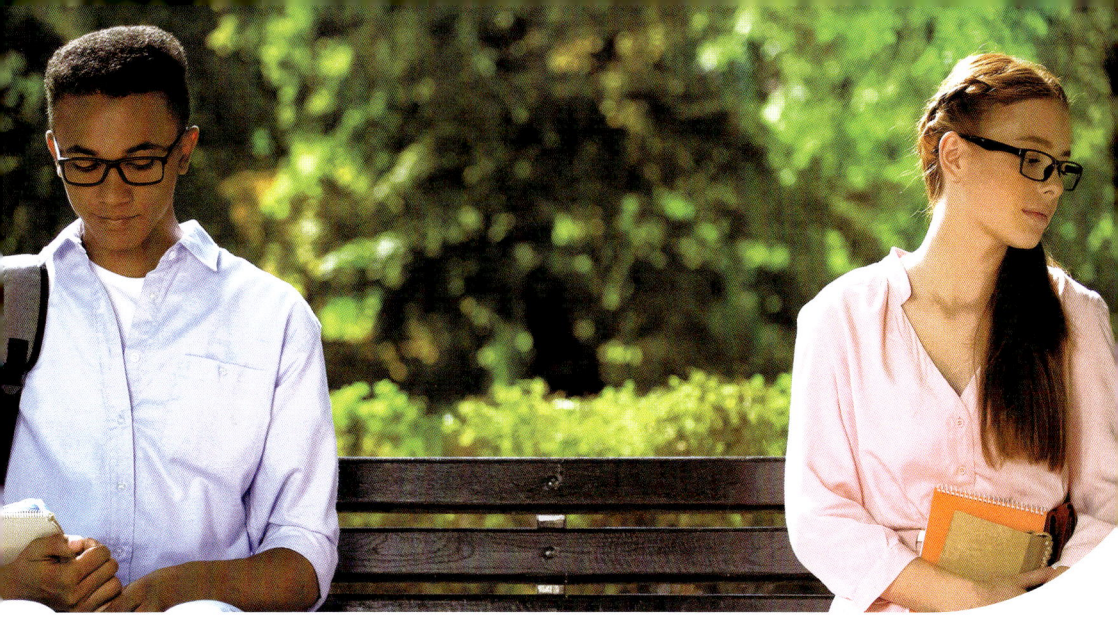

- Cognitive behavioral therapy (CBT) with exposure components is the most effective treatment of SAD for teens. This type of therapy involves slowly and safely confronting the patient's fears.

- Medication that may treat a patient's SAD symptoms is available.

- Support groups are meetings where people with SAD can meet and discuss the condition. These groups may help people with SAD understand their feelings and experiences.

INTRODUCTION

GRIDIRON STAR GRAPPLES WITH SOCIAL ANXIETY

Ricky Williams seemed to have it all. He was a star football player. He had won the Heisman Trophy in 1998. He played football in packed stadiums.

But Williams struggled to do everyday activities. He did not want to leave his house. He started giving interviews to the media in his football helmet. That way he did not have to make eye contact. He even struggled to play outside with his daughter.

In his National Football League (NFL) career, Ricky Williams was a member of the New Orleans Saints, the Miami Dolphins, and the Baltimore Ravens.

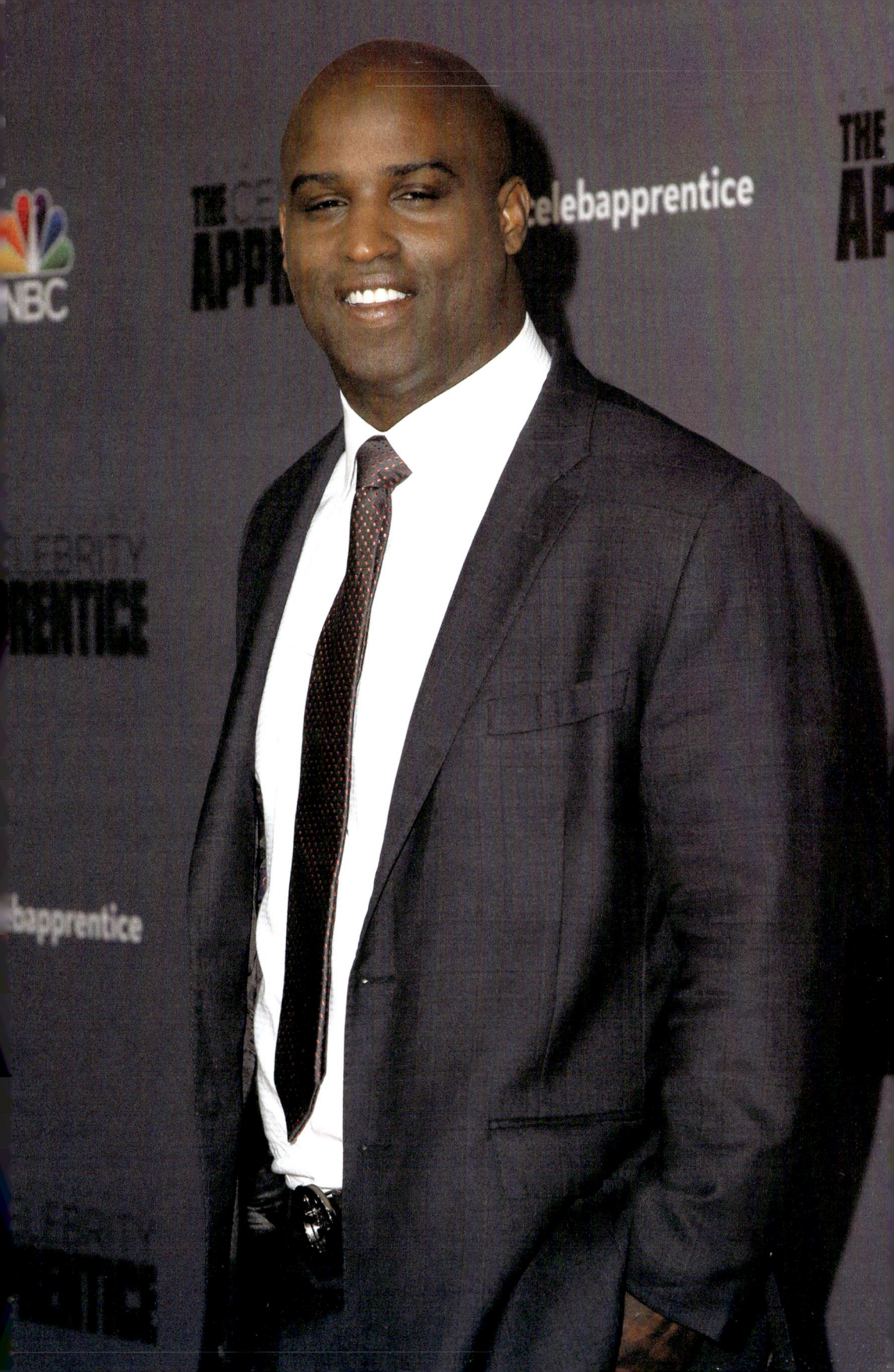

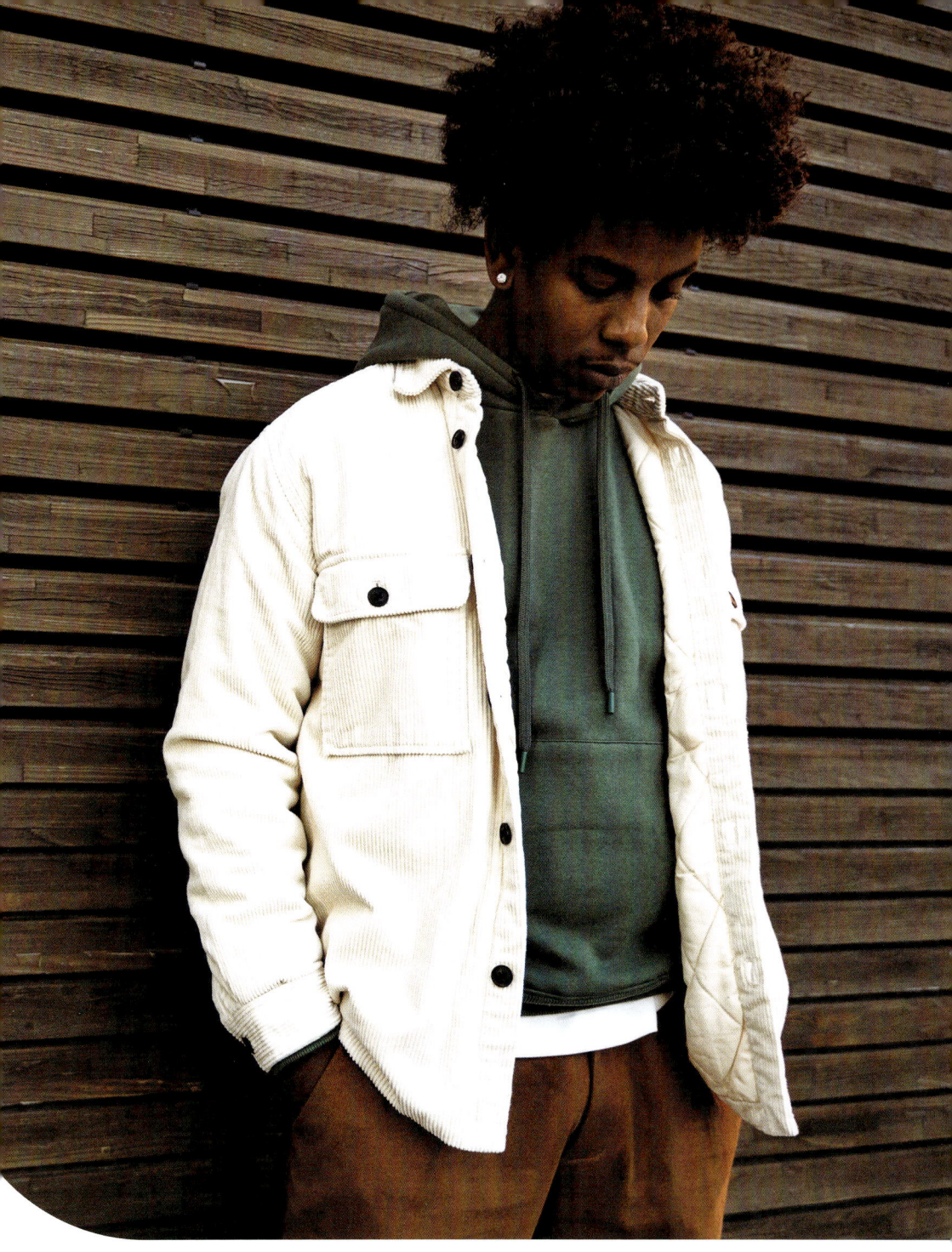

Eye contact can cause feelings of discomfort in people with social anxiety disorder.

Williams did not understand why he had trouble doing these things. He sought help. He says, "I found a therapist and started to educate myself . . . and I started to understand myself."[1] That was how he learned he had social anxiety disorder (SAD). This condition causes an extreme fear of interacting with others. People with SAD typically have trouble performing in front of others. Sports games, presentations, and other social events can cause great distress.

Some people have this condition for years before seeking help. But SAD is very treatable after it is **diagnosed**. Therapists can help people manage the condition. Williams made huge improvements after he started his treatment program. Learning that he had SAD relieved him. He no longer thought there was something wrong with him personally.

HAVING SOCIAL ANXIETY

Many teens have SAD. They might feel anxious when making plans with friends. Getting up in front of the class can be terrifying. Even leaving the house can seem scary. This can lead to **isolation** and loneliness.

But there is help available for teens with this condition. They can learn to manage SAD. It all starts with understanding how SAD works.

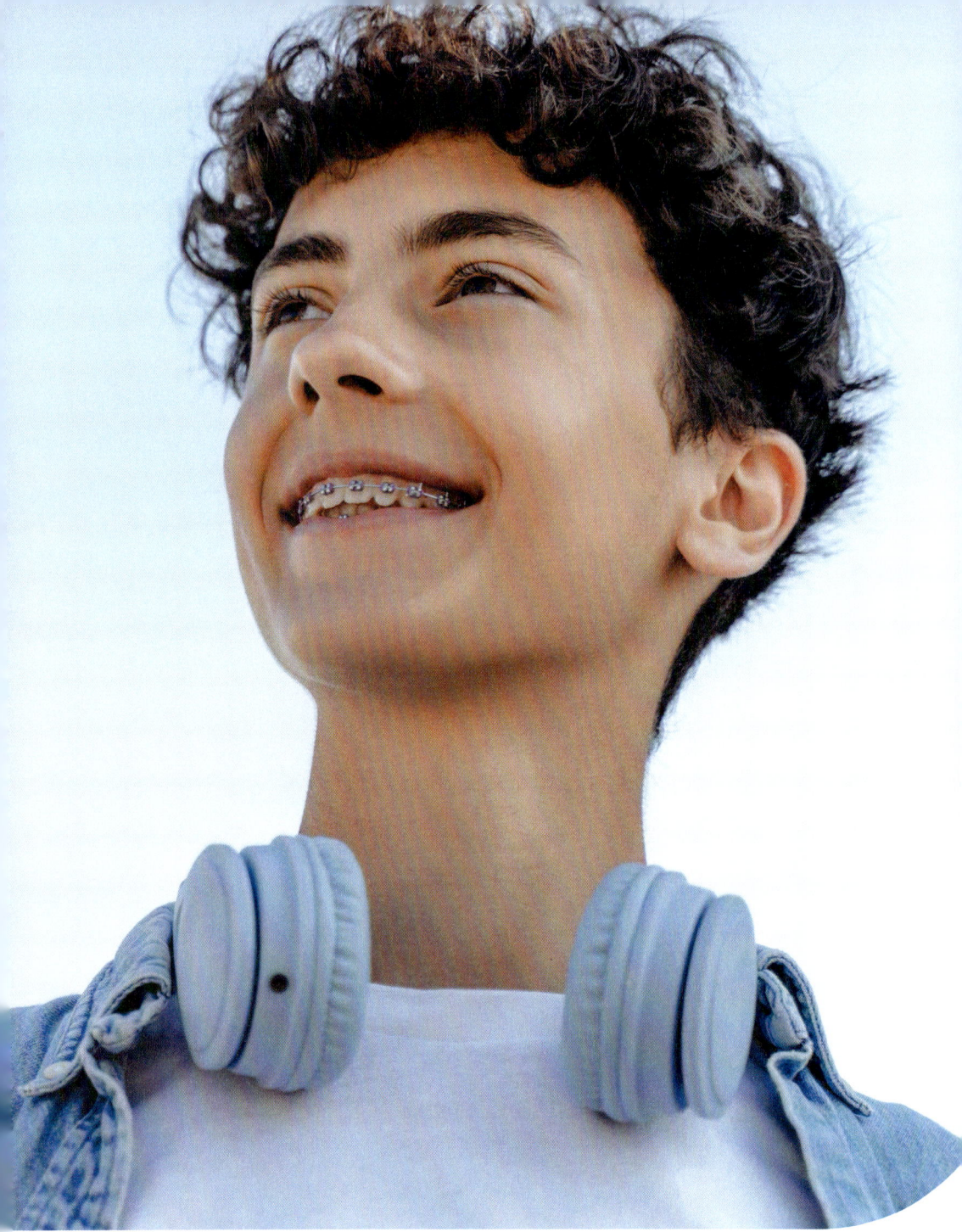

Teens with SAD do not have to suffer quietly. People are there to help.

CHAPTER ONE

WHAT IS SOCIAL ANXIETY?

It is normal for people to sometimes feel shy. But people with SAD are more than simply shy. Everyday social situations can cause them a lot of discomfort. Teens with SAD may avoid friends and family members. They may choose to spend time by themselves instead. This can disrupt teens' lives.

Claire Eastham is a writer with SAD. She began to show signs of the condition when

SAD can affect teens' relationships with their parents, guardians, and caregivers.

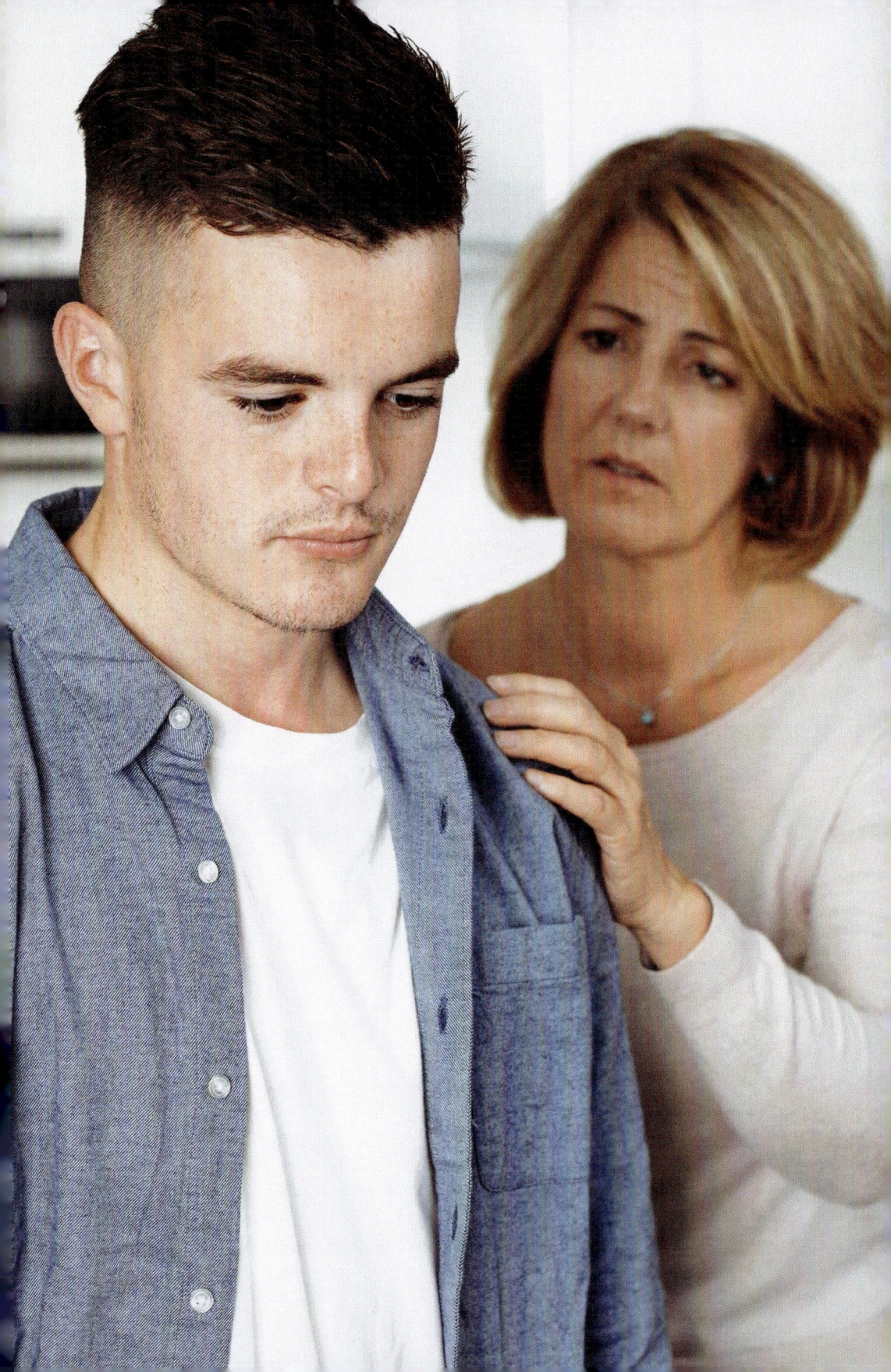

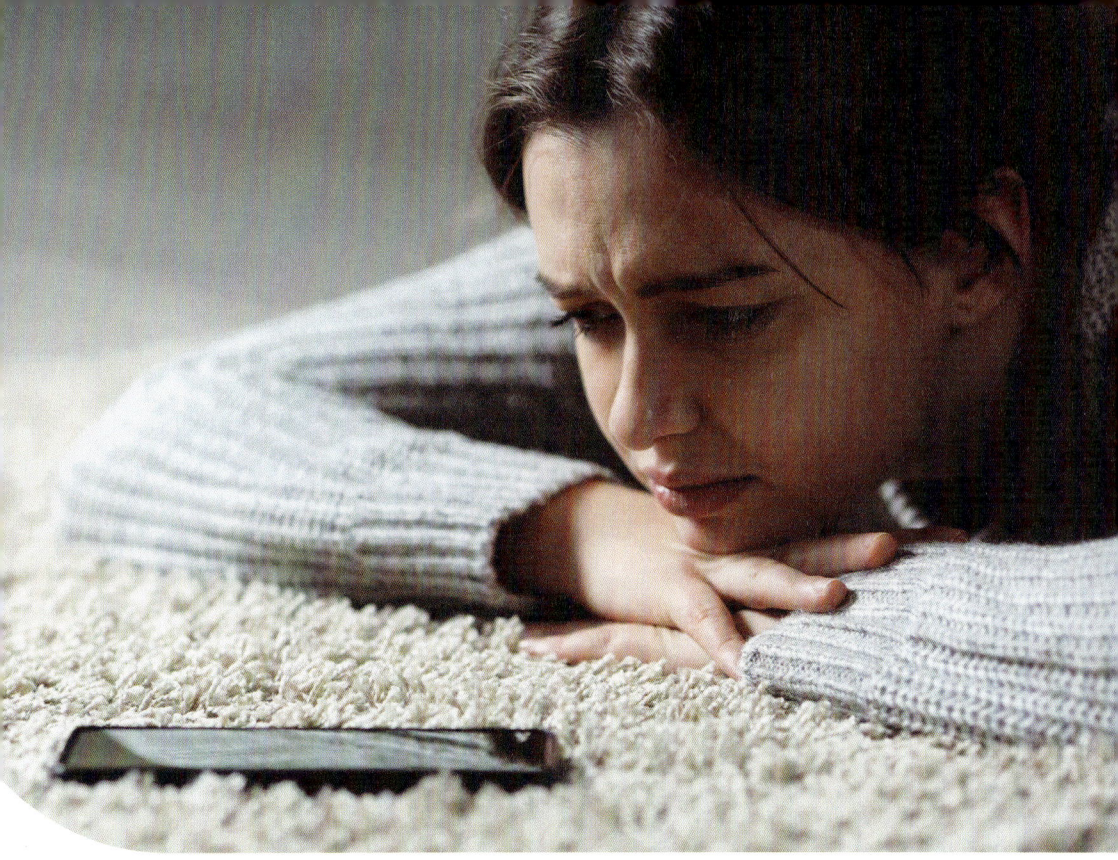

Phone calls are sources of anxiety for some teens with SAD.

she was 6 years old. She went through her teen years before learning she had SAD at 24. She remembers the difficulty her **symptoms** caused her. Being asked to speak in class made her freeze up. When she was alone, she would worry that people thought there was something wrong with her.

WHAT ARE THE SYMPTOMS OF SOCIAL ANXIETY?

People with SAD can experience a range of symptoms. Not everybody with SAD has the same symptoms. And a person with SAD may not experience a given symptom forever. Symptoms may come and go.

Most symptoms of SAD occur in social situations. Any social situation can cause distress. This can include meeting new people. It can also include performing

Who Has Social Anxiety?

More than 15 million adults in the United States have been diagnosed with SAD. About 75 percent of people with SAD developed their first symptoms as a child or a teen. Women are more likely to suffer from SAD than men.

in front of others. Talking on the phone can be difficult as well. So can sharing a meal. SAD can make it hard for teens to speak up in class.

Some symptoms of SAD are physical. These symptoms can resemble panic. A person's heart might start to beat faster. The person may breathe rapidly. Their muscles may tighten. They might also start to blush and sweat. Their mind may go blank. These symptoms can be frightening and tiring.

Sometimes the sense of panic is more severe. A panic attack is a sudden spell of intense fear. They can occur when there is not a real cause for panic. Panic attacks can cause strong physical symptoms. These include chest pain. They also include

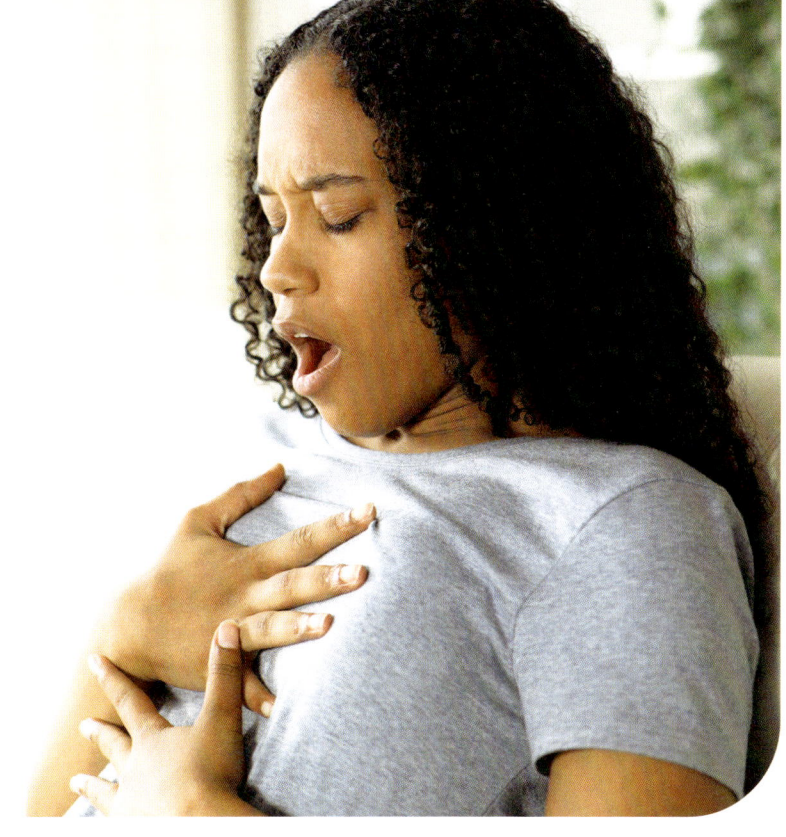

Anybody, including people without diagnosed mental health conditions, can have a panic attack.

difficulty breathing. A rapid heart rate may also occur. Sometimes people having panic attacks worry that they are dying. The symptoms can be that powerful.

Social situations can cause panic attacks in people with SAD. The attacks can add to a person's fears. A teen with SAD may have a panic attack during a school presentation. This can cause them to avoid presenting in the future.

SAD may also produce many emotional and mental symptoms. People with SAD may worry a lot about being embarrassed. They may worry that other people will notice their anxiety. And they may have

People with SAD tend to perceive certain social situations as more embarrassing than people without SAD.

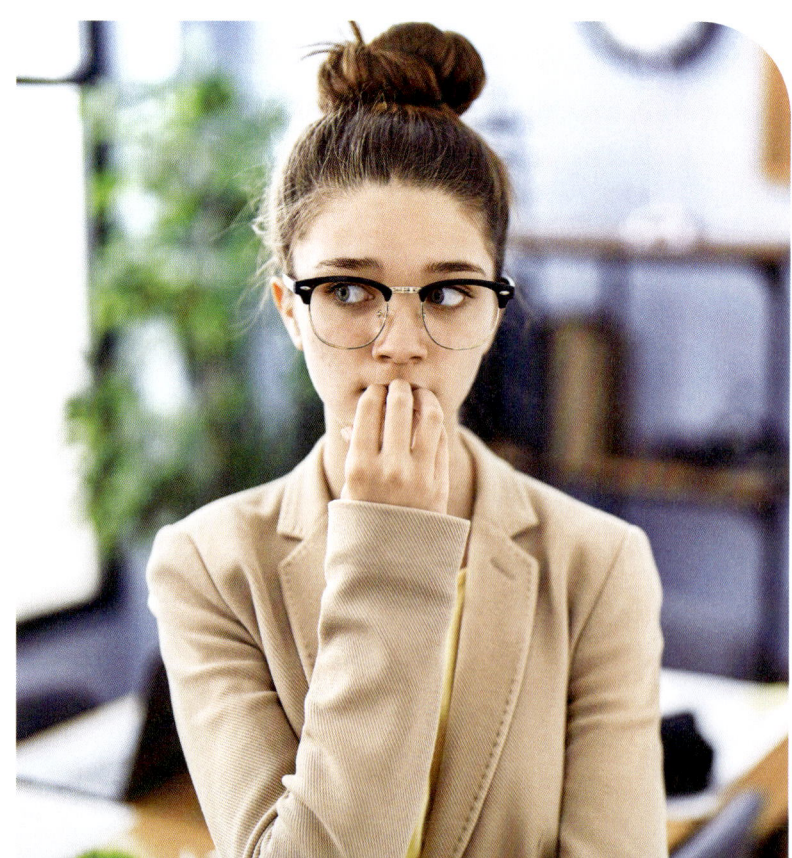

negative expectations when entering a social situation.

Sometimes a person with SAD imagines threats that are not there. Researchers spoke with young people with SAD about their symptoms. One 12-year-old talked about their fear that other people were making fun of them. They said, "There were these three girls laughing, and I thought they were laughing at me."[2] A person without SAD may not have made this assumption.

A person with SAD does not need to be around other people to have symptoms. They may **ruminate** on memories of social situations. They may painstakingly examine their actions. Any flaws they find may cause them distress. These feelings can cause people with SAD to avoid social situations altogether.

WHAT CAUSES SOCIAL ANXIETY?

SAD does not have one simple cause. It likely has several causes that combine to make developing the condition more likely. Some of these causes are biological. These include the traits a person inherits from their parents. They also include a person's brain structure. Other causes are environmental. A person's experiences may make them more likely to develop SAD.

 Research has shown that a person's genetic traits affect their chances of developing SAD. Genetics is the study of inherited traits. People inherit traits from their parents. These traits are passed down

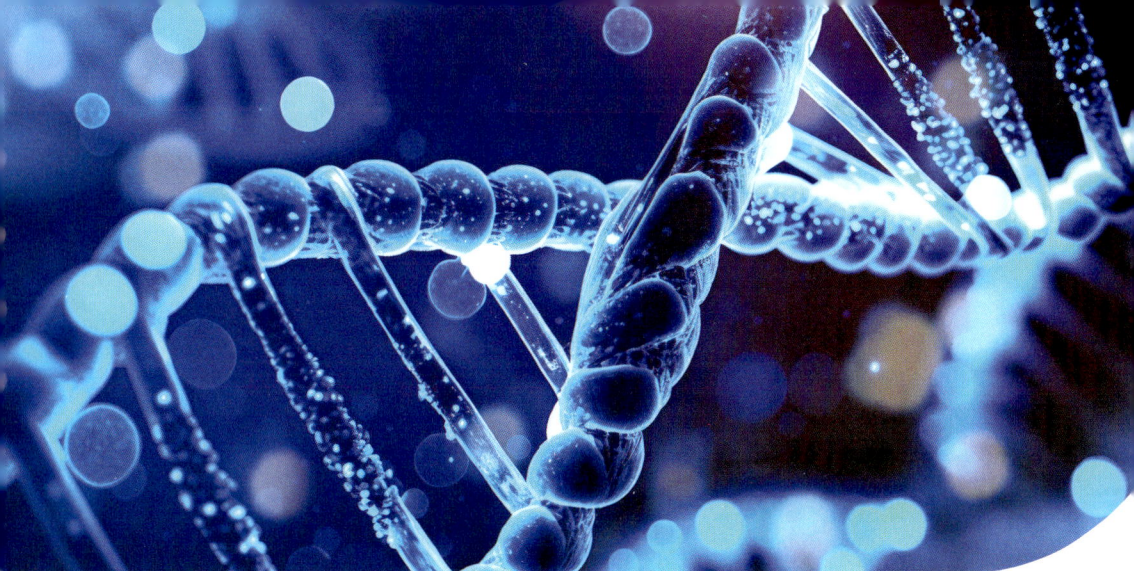

Sections of genetic material are called genes. The combination of several genes can produce complex traits in people.

through the genetic material in people's bodies. Some genetic material may make a person more likely to develop SAD.

Studies of twins have led researchers to suspect that the cause of SAD is partly genetic. In twin studies, researchers examine identical and fraternal twins. Identical twins share almost all of their genetic material. Fraternal twins share only half. Researchers begin by assuming that SAD's causes are not genetic. This would mean pairs of fraternal and identical twins should develop SAD at similar rates. But studies show that this is not the case. Identical twins are more likely to develop SAD together than fraternal twins are. Researchers point to genetics as the cause.

Identical twins occur in about 3 to 5 births out of every 1,000.

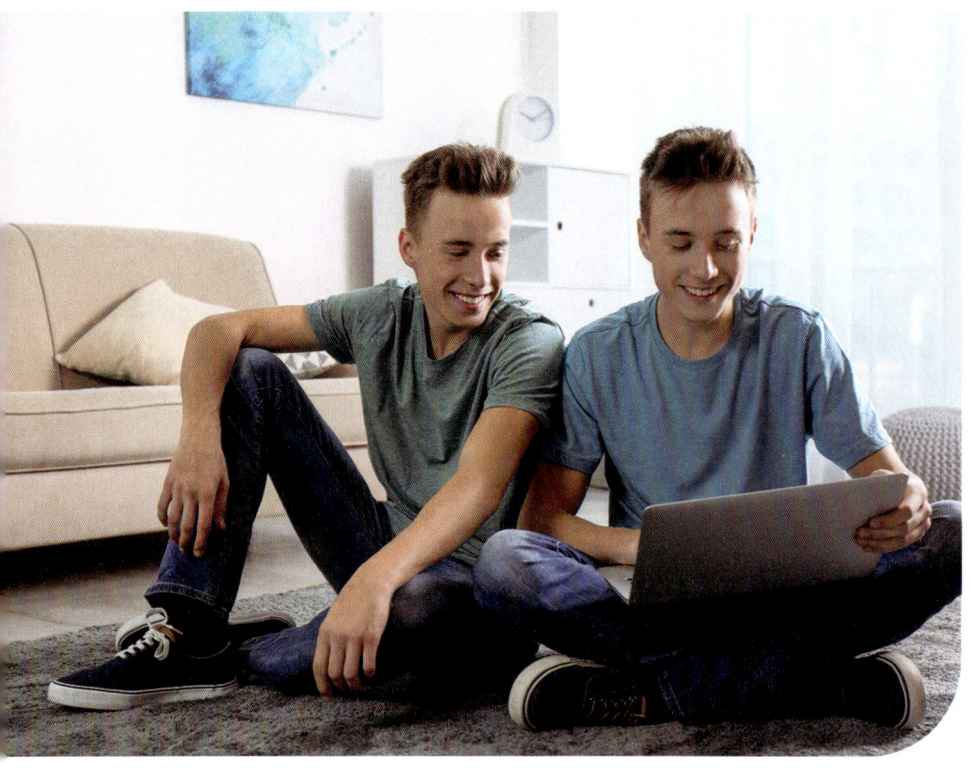

The structure of a person's brain can also be related to SAD. Studies have shown that people with SAD are more likely to possess certain brain features. These include increased activity in parts of the brain linked to fear. One of these parts is called the amygdala. This part plays a role in people's responses to threats.

ENVIRONMENTAL CAUSES

A person's chances of developing SAD may be related to early interactions with parents or caregivers. One theory of childhood development explains how this could work. The theory holds that babies form attachment styles with their caregivers. These styles form due to how caregivers interact with the baby.

An attachment style can affect the way a person bonds with others as an adult.

One attachment style is called insecure attachment. Babies form this style when they are not confident their caregivers will comfort them. People who grow up with this style may struggle to feel confident in their adult relationships. Some studies have shown that having an insecure attachment style may make a person more likely to develop SAD.

Parenting methods as children grow up can also affect a person's chances of developing SAD. Studies have connected harsh parenting with the development of SAD in children. A lack of affection from caregivers can also raise a child's

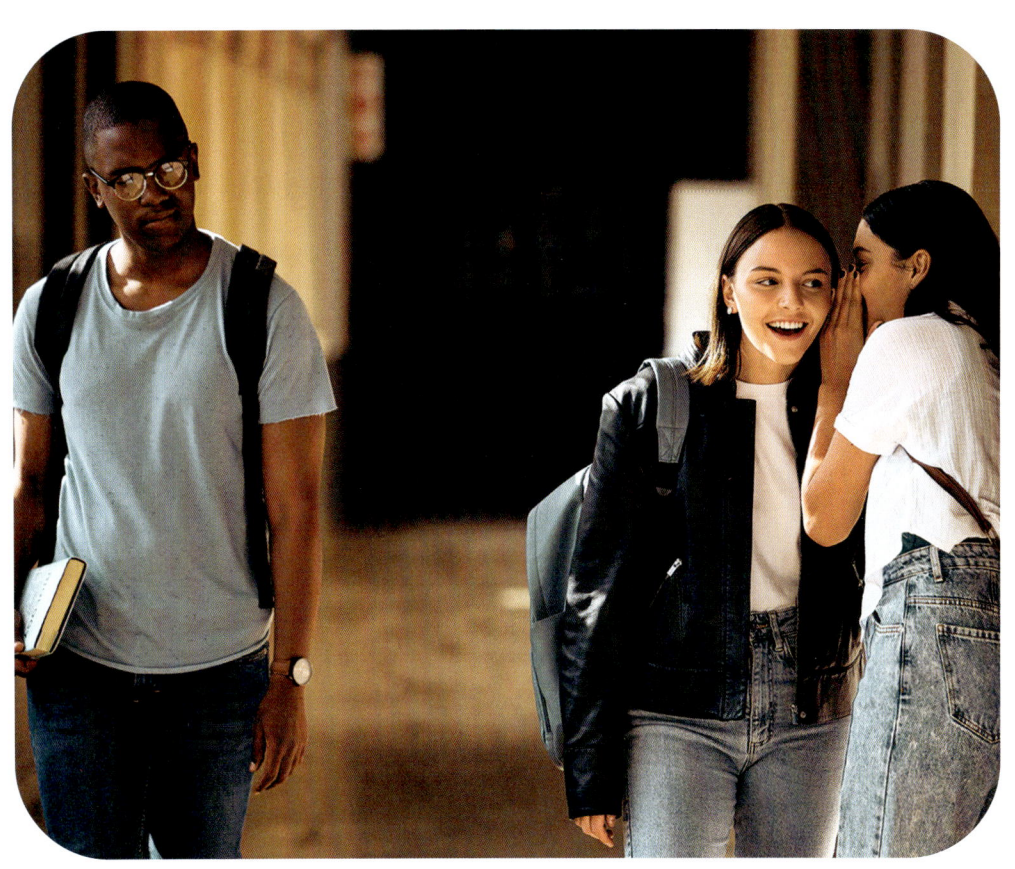

About 20 percent of students in the United States report having been bullied.

chances of SAD. So can an overcontrolling parenting style.

Being bullied has also been linked to SAD. Teens who are bullied are more likely to develop the condition. The condition can persist even after the bullying has stopped.

CHAPTER TWO

EFFECTS OF SOCIAL ANXIETY

SAD can greatly affect a teen's social life. Teens with SAD can struggle to make friends. They might also be uncomfortable playing sports. And they might not want to go to school.

SAD can cause young people to feel shy when meeting new people. It might also cause people to limit their social activities. Teens might not join a club they are interested in. They may find ways to

Raising one's hand in class can be difficult for teens with SAD.

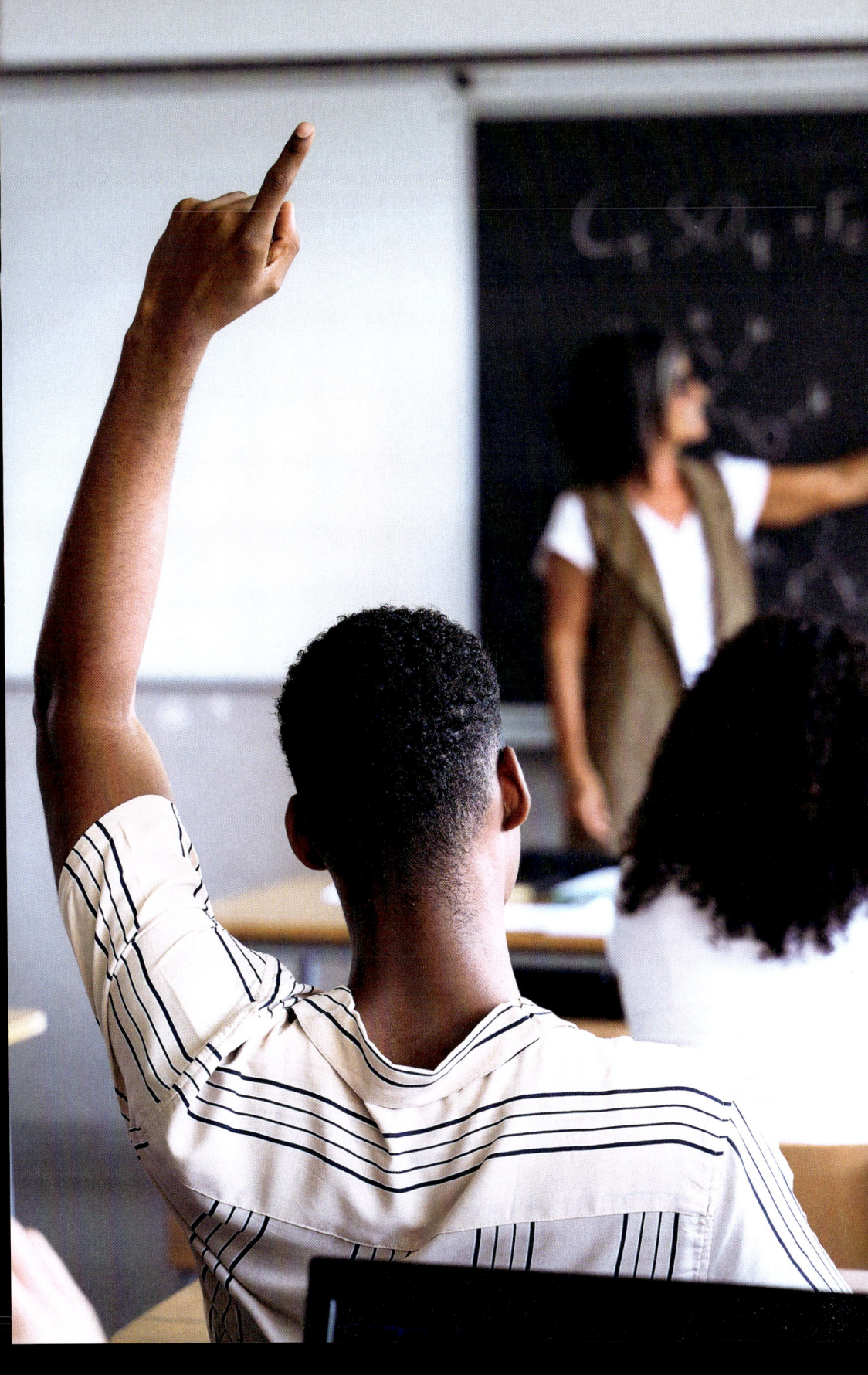

avoid conversations. One 12-year-old said, "I will try to look busy, . . . go on my phone, [or] try to look away."[3]

Teens with SAD may also struggle to date. They may avoid romantic relationships even if they want them. They may decline dates. They may not attend school dances. This can cause feelings of loneliness.

SOCIAL ANXIETY AND SCHOOL

SAD can affect more parts of a teen's life than their friendships. Teens with the condition can also struggle in school. SAD can cause teens to fear speaking up in class. They might also not have the confidence to give presentations. Some teens might not feel comfortable asking a teacher for help.

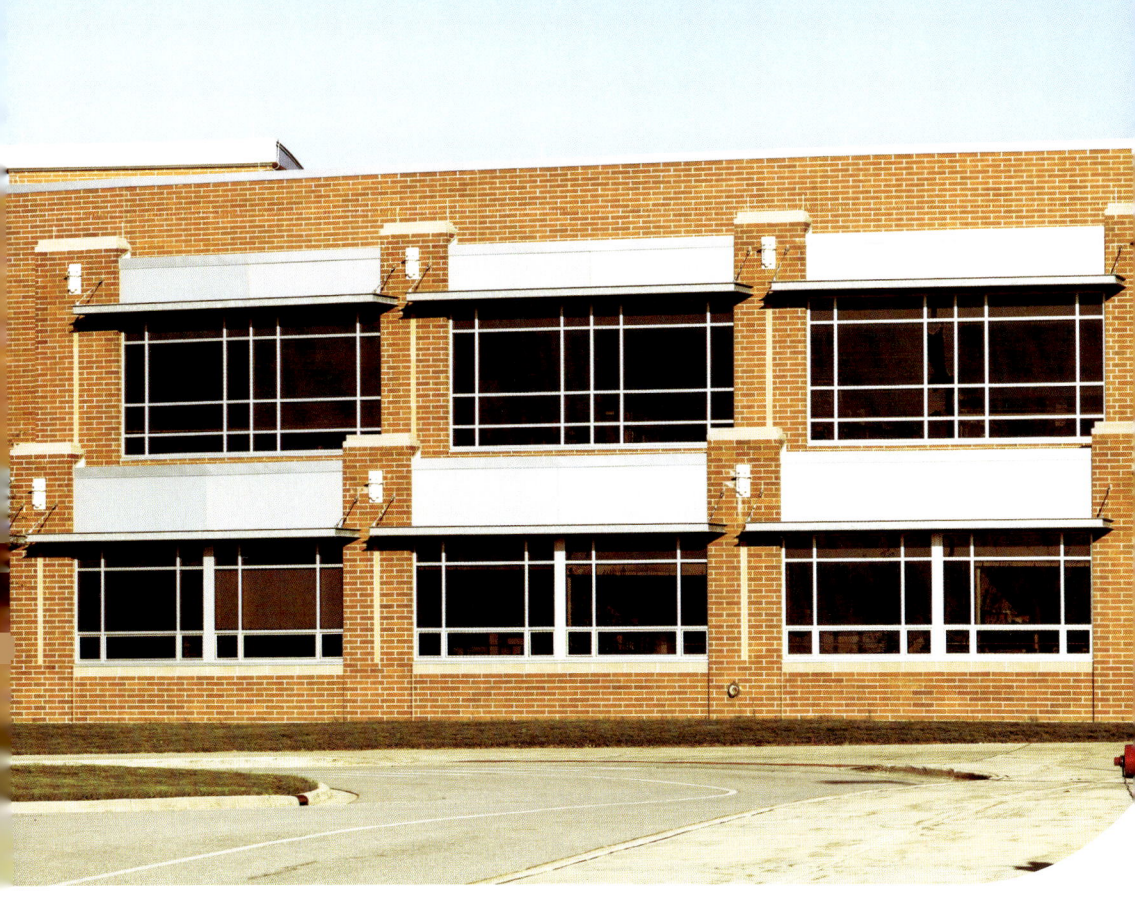

For many teens with SAD, school is a significant source of anxiety.

SAD can result in lower grades. Students may be marked down for not participating in class. They might also not do their part in group projects. This can eventually lead to more severe outcomes. These include failing classes. Mehek Azra is a teen with SAD. She explains, "You'd rather get a zero than participate because you are afraid your classmates will secretly laugh at you."[4]

Zoe is another teen with SAD who feels its effects at school. She would have stomachaches on school mornings. Her anxiety caused these and

Job interviews can be nerve-racking for teens with SAD. Practicing the interview beforehand with a friend or family member may help reduce anxiety.

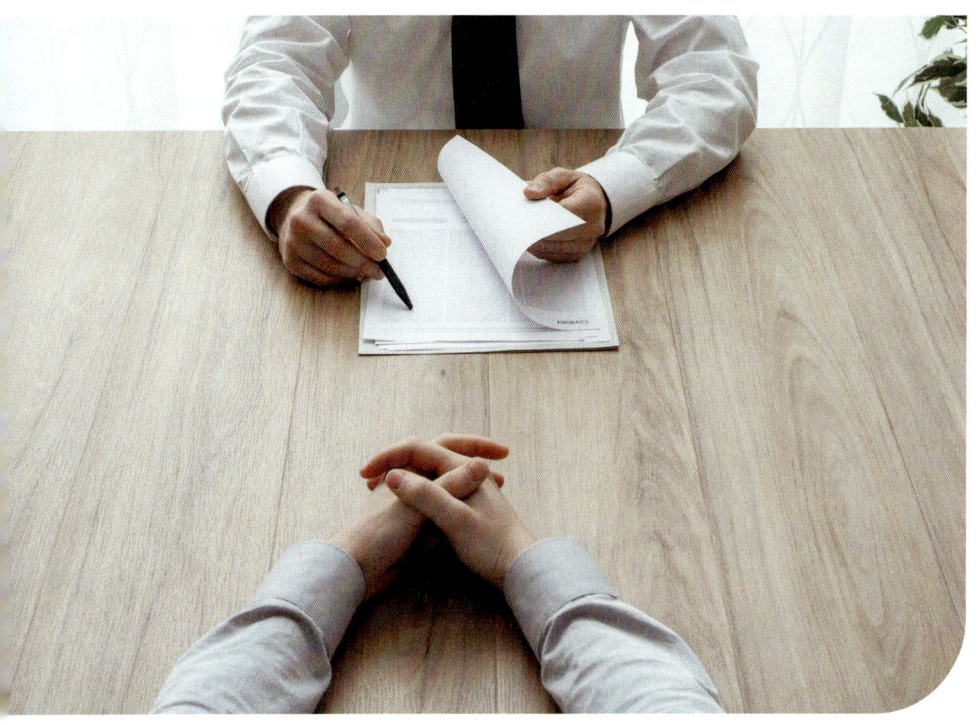

other symptoms. Zoe's mother explains what would happen when she would drop off her daughter. She says, "[Zoe] would get dressed, pack her bag, and drive with me to school. However, she could not move once at the entrance."[5]

OTHER CHALLENGES OF SOCIAL ANXIETY

SAD can affect a teen's life outside of school. Many teens apply for part-time jobs. But teens with SAD may struggle to get these jobs. Interviews can cause a lot of anxiety. Teens may worry about their performance in job interviews. This may cause them to avoid job opportunities.

Teens with SAD may have low self-esteem. Self-esteem is how people feel about themselves. SAD can make people feel like they are worthless. Having few friends due to SAD can also cause low self-esteem. So can struggling in school.

Sophie is a young adult with SAD. She remembers having low self-esteem as a teen. She felt as if there was something wrong with the way she looked. She worried that other people felt the same way about her. Walking into a room was very hard. She felt as if other people were judging her appearance as soon as she entered.

Teens with SAD may have a higher chance of developing other mental health conditions. They are at a higher risk of developing depression. They are also more likely to develop unsafe substance use.

CELEBRITIES WITH SOCIAL ANXIETY

Naomi Osaka, Tennis Player

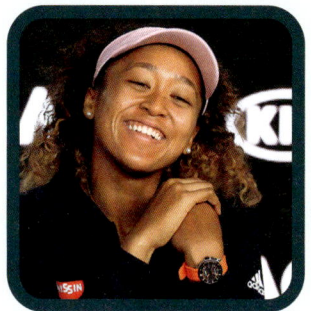

"Anyone that has seen me at tournaments will notice that I'm often wearing headphones as that helps dull my social anxiety."

Source: Quoted in Sarah Ellis, "What It's Like to Be a Celebrity with Social Anxiety Disorder," HealthCentral, *June 8, 2021. www.healthcentral.com.*

Cole Sprouse, Actor

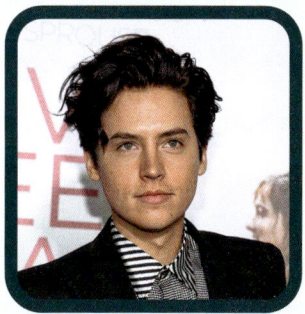

"My social anxiety feels a lot like sitting in a sauna when it's just a bit too hot."

Source: Quoted in "Cole Sprouse Opens Up About His Struggles with Social Anxiety," YouTube, *uploaded by The Diary of a CEO Clips. www.youtube.com.*

Shailene Woodley, Actress

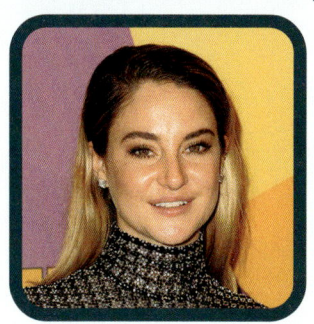

"I had extreme social anxiety—I never felt safe, I never felt like I could trust people, I never felt like it was okay to not be in control."

Source: Quoted in Nojan Aminosharei, "Shailene Woodley Gets Personal About Coping with Anxiety in the Time of COVID-19," Harper's Bazaar, *May 12, 2020. www.harpersbazaar.com.*

Many celebrities suffer from SAD. Here are three celebrities' experiences with the condition in their own words.

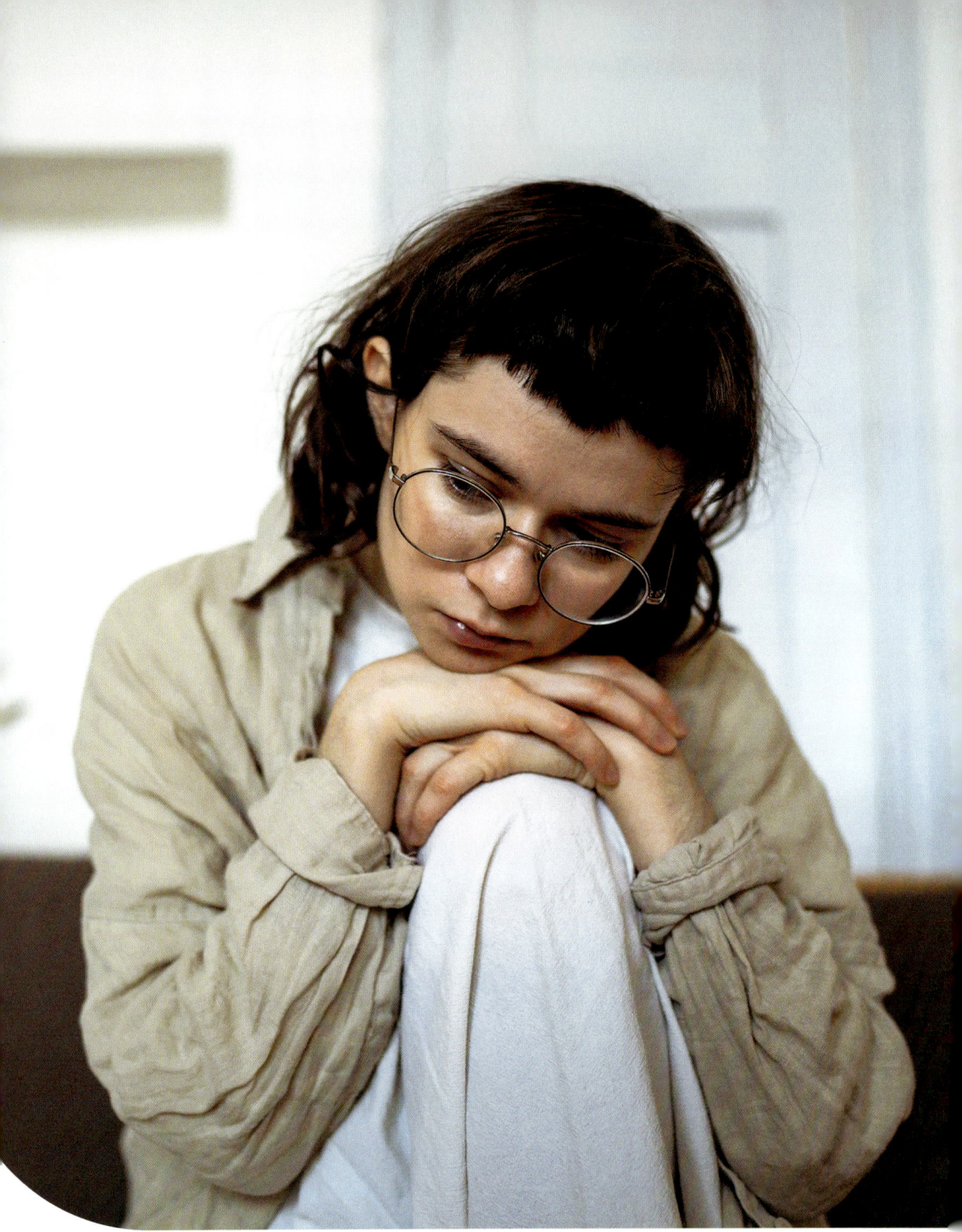

About 20 percent of teens in the United States have had an episode of depression.

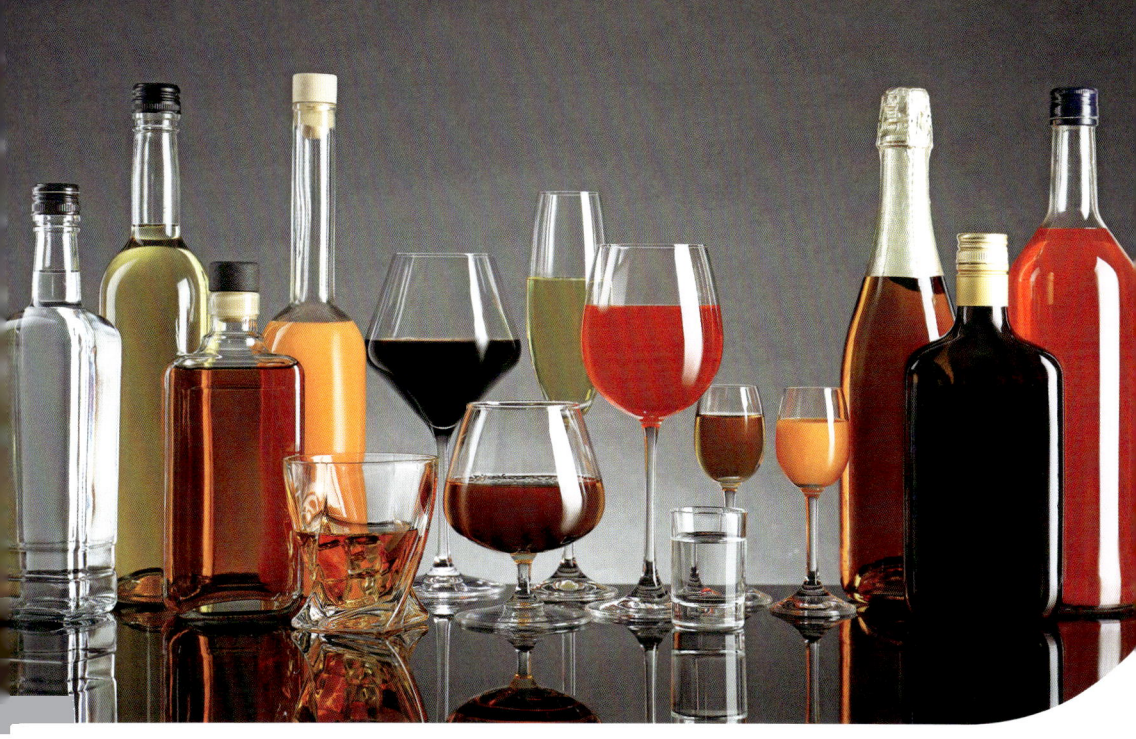

A 2023 study found that 33.1 percent of people in the United States between the ages of 12 and 20 have had at least one drink in their lives.

About 20 percent of people with SAD have alcohol dependence.

Cynthia Kipp first felt SAD symptoms as a child. She began drinking alcohol when she was a teen to cope. The alcohol helped her relax around other people. But she eventually lost control of her drinking. Kipp found a healthier way to deal with her SAD as an adult. She got therapy. She also

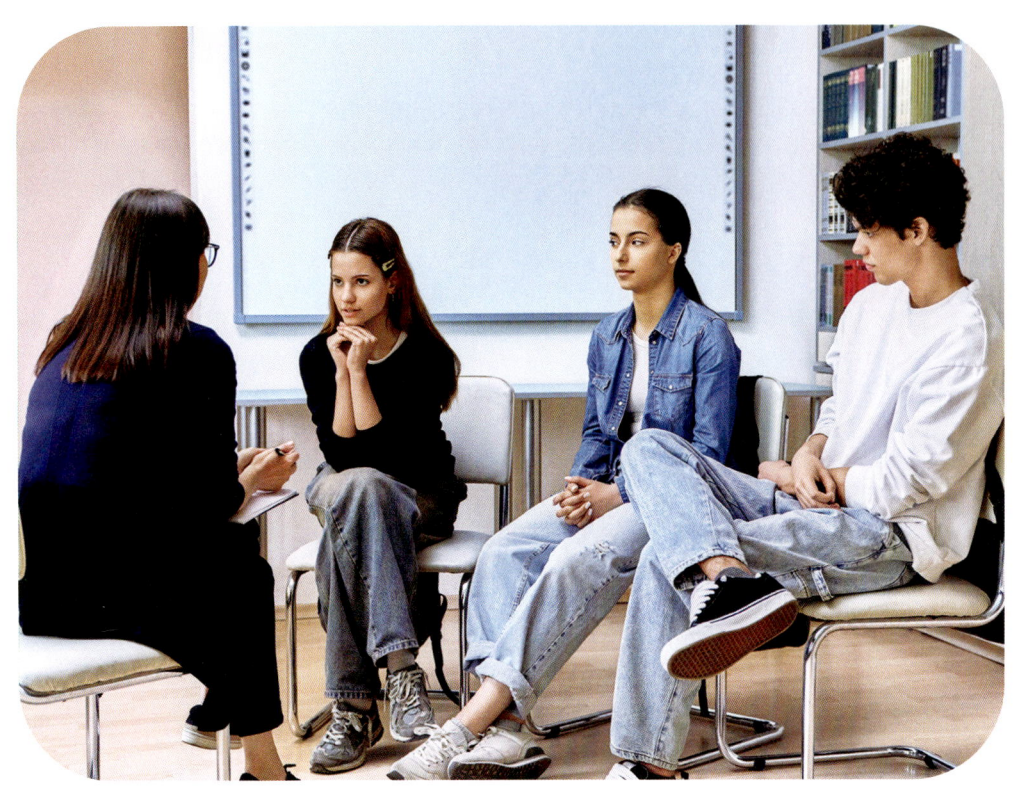

Group therapy is one treatment option for alcohol addiction.

attended support meetings for people with alcohol addiction.

Some people with SAD develop suicidal thoughts. It is unclear whether SAD causes suicidal thoughts. But studies have shown that having SAD can make a person more likely to think about or attempt suicide. Researchers have considered explanations

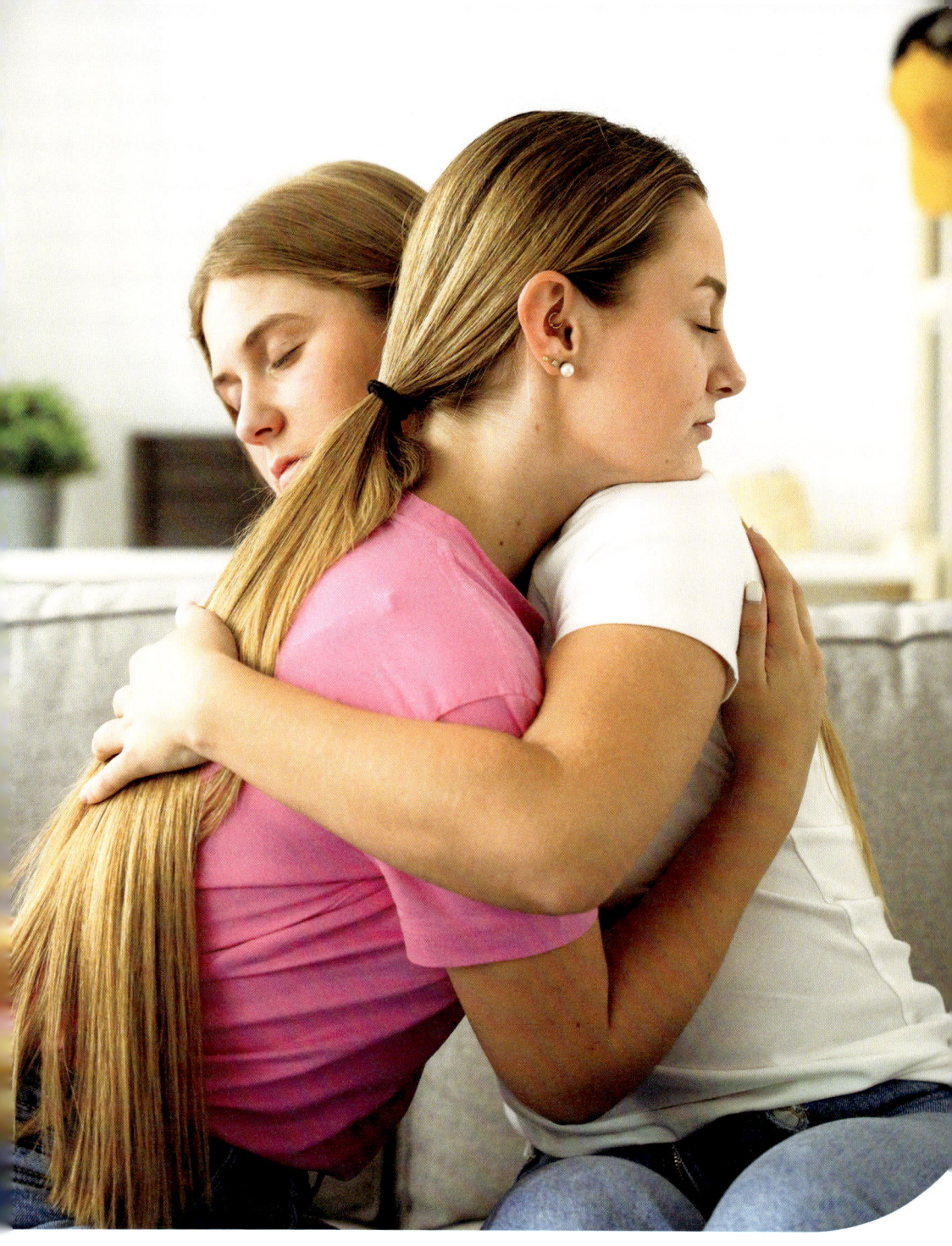

Talking about suicide does not raise a person's risk of suicide. It may actually reduce the risk of suicide.

for this relationship. The negative feelings that SAD can cause may lead some to consider suicide. SAD can also cause people to isolate themselves. This can make finding support for suicidal thoughts difficult.

Hilary had endured her SAD for years before she knew she had it. She would avoid the situations that scared her. She would refuse to use public restrooms even when she needed to. And she hated the idea of going to the grocery store by herself. Her self-esteem began to fall. Her mental health worsened. She says, "I started to feel like I had no place in society and that I was a waste of space. I started to have thoughts of suicide."[6] She recognized the danger of these thoughts. She sought out emergency health care.

That was how Hilary learned she had SAD. She began to receive treatment and support. She made progress in her mental health. Her treatment involved slowly confronting her fears. Social situations that used to scare her no longer did. She says that she is grateful that she asked for help.

Shyness or Social Anxiety?

Some symptoms of SAD can resemble shyness. But there are key differences. Shyness is a personality trait. It does not require treatment. Being shy does not seriously reduce a person's quality of life. SAD is a mental health condition that requires treatment. Its symptoms affect people's ability to live their lives.

CHAPTER THREE

FINDING SUPPORT FOR SOCIAL ANXIETY

There are treatments available to teens with SAD. Therapy can help teens deal with their anxiety in many cases. Medication can also help. Other forms of support include support groups. These treatments can help teens with SAD cope with the condition. **Psychologist** Kathryn D. Boger says, "When kids get appropriate treatment for anxiety, it can make an enormous difference in the **trajectory** of their lives."[7]

Treatment for SAD can help teens with the condition feel more comfortable in social situations.

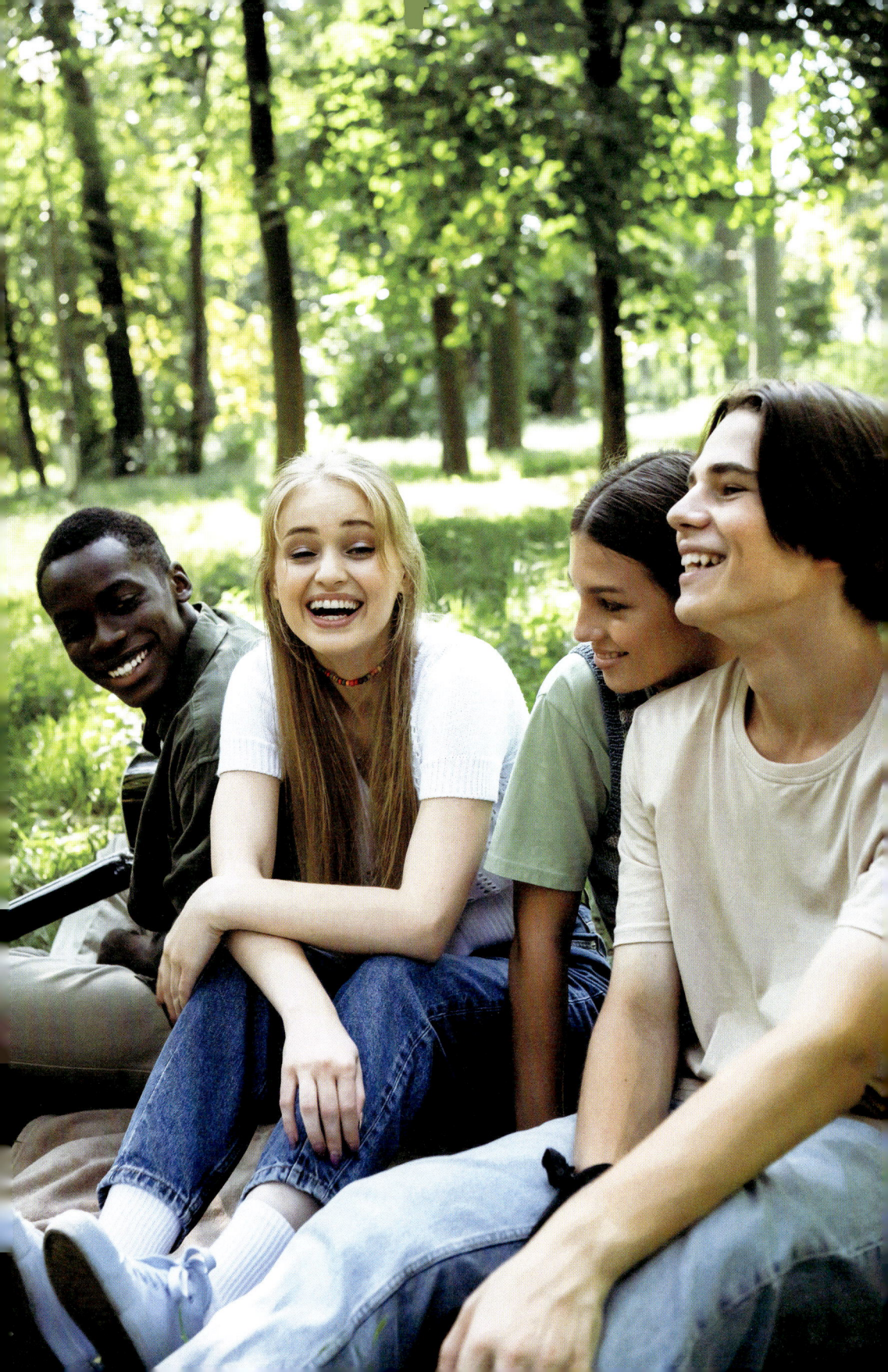

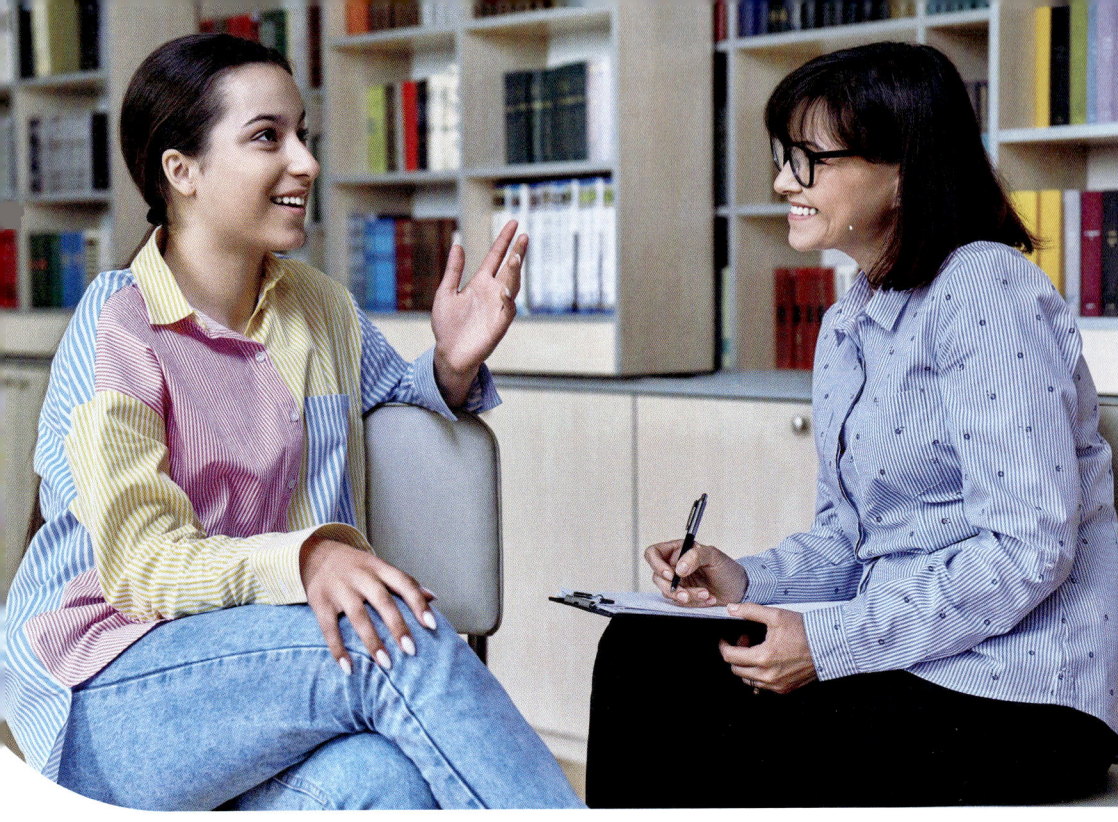

School counselors have a duty to support the development of students. They work with students to address concerns about mental health.

Teens should seek help if they think they have SAD. They can tell their parents or trusted adults about their symptoms. Teens can also talk to their teachers and school counselors. These authority figures can connect teens with mental health care professionals. Teens can talk about their concerns with doctors as well.

THERAPY

Therapy is often used to treat SAD. There are different kinds of therapists. These include psychologists and **psychiatrists**. They include counselors and certain kinds of social workers as well. There are also different kinds of therapy. Some are better suited to treat certain mental health conditions than others.

Certain forms of **cognitive** behavioral therapy (CBT) are the most effective treatments for teens with SAD. In CBT, a patient typically meets with a therapist for weekly sessions. These sessions may continue for up to 20 weeks. CBT aims to help teens with SAD gradually and safely confront their fears. Therapists are often seen as coaches who also help teach their patients skills. These skills include recognizing negative thoughts. They also include problem solving. Being aware of one's feelings is another taught skill.

Studies have found that between 58 and 75 percent of CBT patients see a reduction in symptoms. Ramani Durvasula is a psychologist. She explains the benefits of CBT. She says, "If you can help a person change how they think . . . about a situation, you'll likely change the reactions and the behaviors."[8]

There are different kinds of CBT. Some are more effective for teens with SAD than others. Research has shown that teens with SAD benefit most from forms of CBT that involve exposure therapy. Exposure therapy allows patients to safely confront their fears.

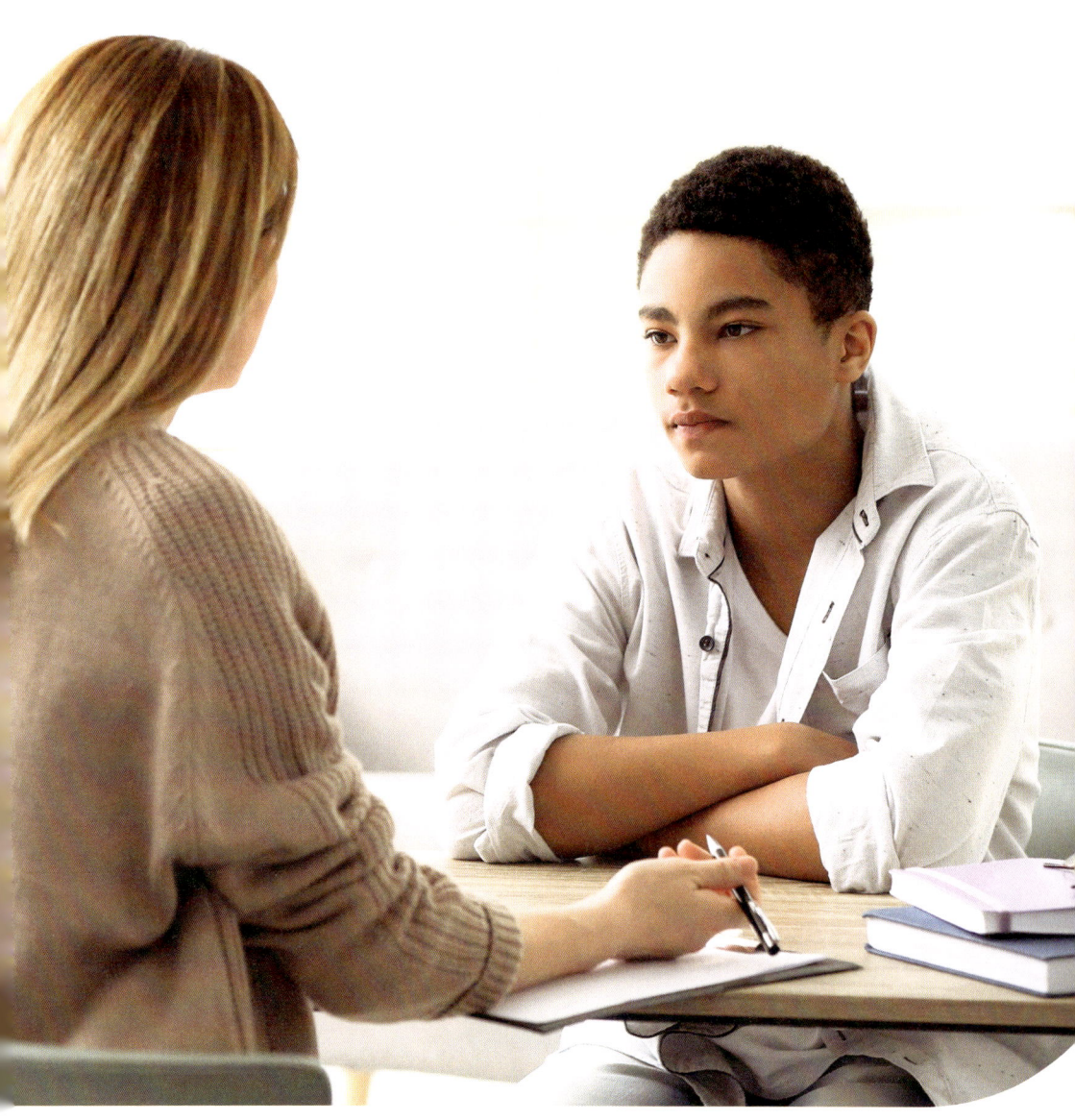

Some therapists specialize in treating mental health conditions in teens.

People naturally avoid what they fear. But this avoidance can make their fears worse. Exposure therapy can show a person that what they fear is not as scary as they think. This may reduce anxiety symptoms.

Exposure therapy slowly exposes a patient to their fears. The therapist works with the patient to make a list of fears to overcome. Then the therapist usually starts gently. They may ask the patient to confront their smallest fear. This helps build confidence. The patient may then be ready to tackle larger challenges. A patient with SAD may start by texting a new friend. The therapy may end with the patient signing up to perform in a school play.

Eleanor Segall struggled with several mental health conditions as a teen. She had

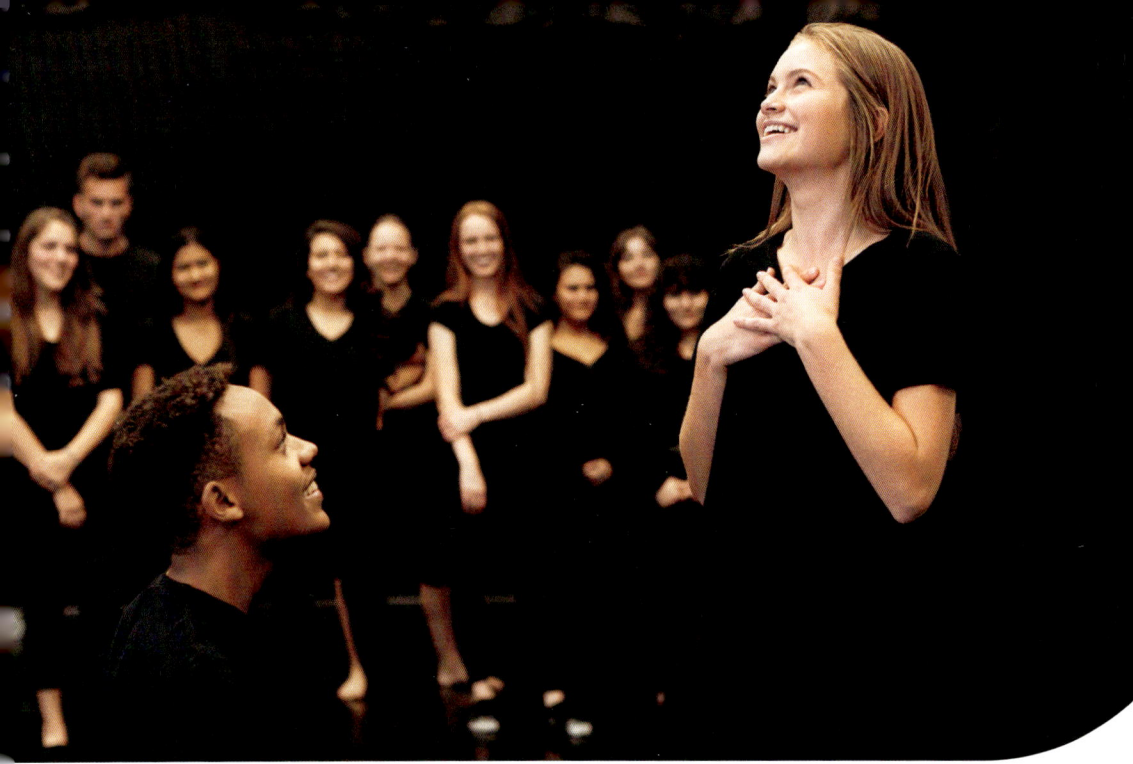

Treatment can help teens with SAD pursue their interests.

to go to the hospital. This made her worry about fitting in with her peers. Soon she developed SAD. She was afraid that other people were judging her. She describes how her SAD lowered her self-esteem. She avoided parties and other gatherings.

Eleanor eventually got help for her SAD. She opened up about her symptoms to her friends and family. And she began to

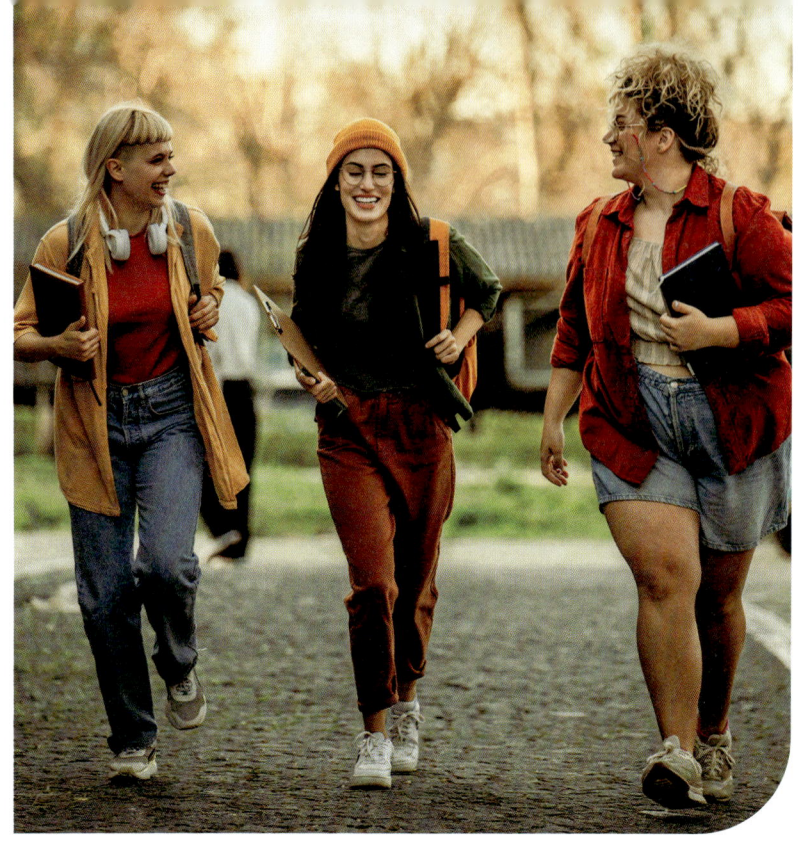

Social skills training can help patients strengthen their conversational skills.

receive CBT. She talks about the support she received. Her loved ones would help her complete her exposure tasks. With Eleanor's permission, her parents would take her on drives. Her friends would visit her at her house. This exposure helped her handle situations she used to fear more strongly.

Chris Rentfrow can remember struggling with SAD as a teen. He describes how hard he was on himself. He wanted to be a perfect athlete and student. Everyday moments of embarrassment caused him distress. He suffered for years without getting help. But he eventually decided to get CBT. He says that it helped him take control of his SAD.

Social Skills Training

A person with SAD may struggle to use their social skills. Their anxiety can keep them from behaving as they want to. This can then further encourage the person to avoid social situations. Social skills training (SST) is a treatment that can help. A therapist practicing SST helps patients develop and use social skills.

MEDICATION

Medication can help reduce SAD symptoms. Health-care providers prescribe different kinds of medication for SAD. Selective serotonin reuptake inhibitors (SSRIs) are among the most common. Serotonin is a chemical that the body's nerves use to communicate. The chemical plays several roles in the brain. Research has connected serotonin with mood.

SSRIs affect how nerves use serotonin. Nerves normally absorb this chemical. But SSRIs block this absorption. This causes serotonin to build up in the brain. SSRIs may reduce symptoms of some mental health conditions. These conditions include SAD. SSRIs may also make therapy for SAD more effective. It may take weeks

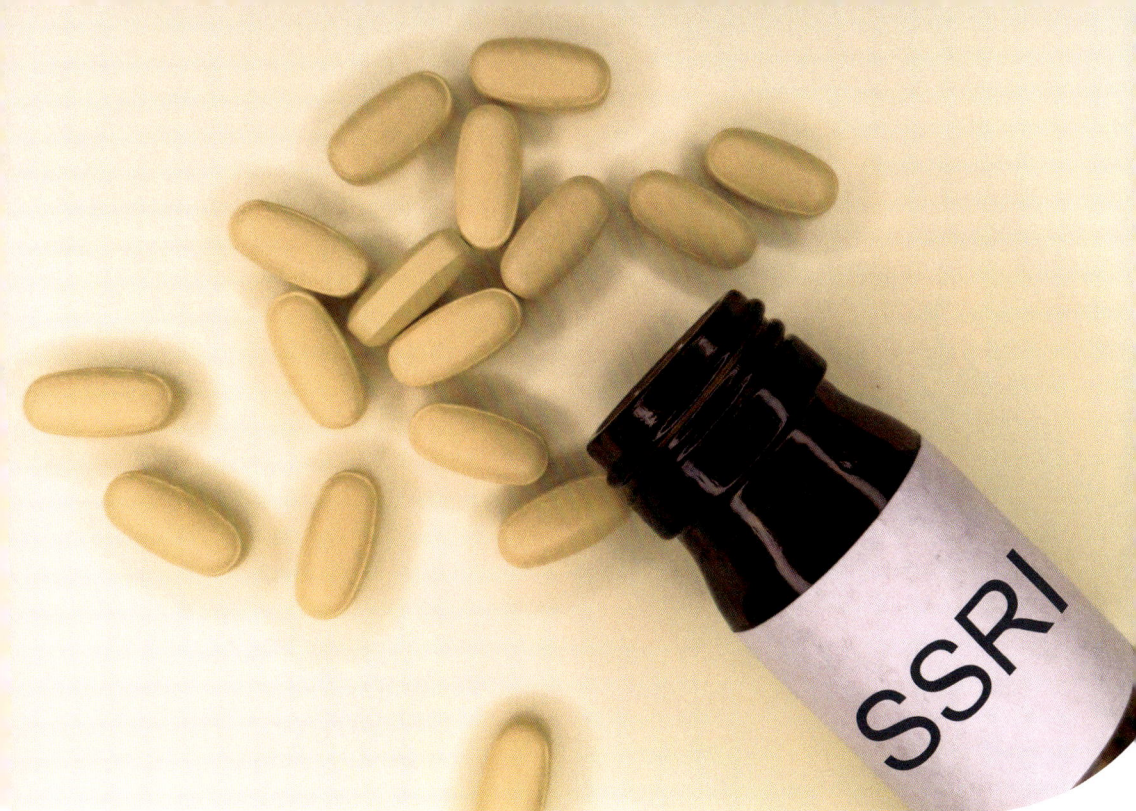

SSRIs are usually given to patients in the form of pills.

or months for a person on SSRIs to notice a change.

SSRIs can have side effects. These are effects that differ from the desired effect of a medication. Side effects of SSRIs include changes in weight. Dry mouth is also common. Sometimes SSRIs can make anxiety worse. A person's side effects may go away as they continue to take a medicine. But some medications may not be a good fit for a person. People taking SSRIs are often asked to regularly check in with a health care professional. That way they can discuss any concerns they have.

Attending a support group is not a treatment for SAD, but it can be useful when combined with treatment.

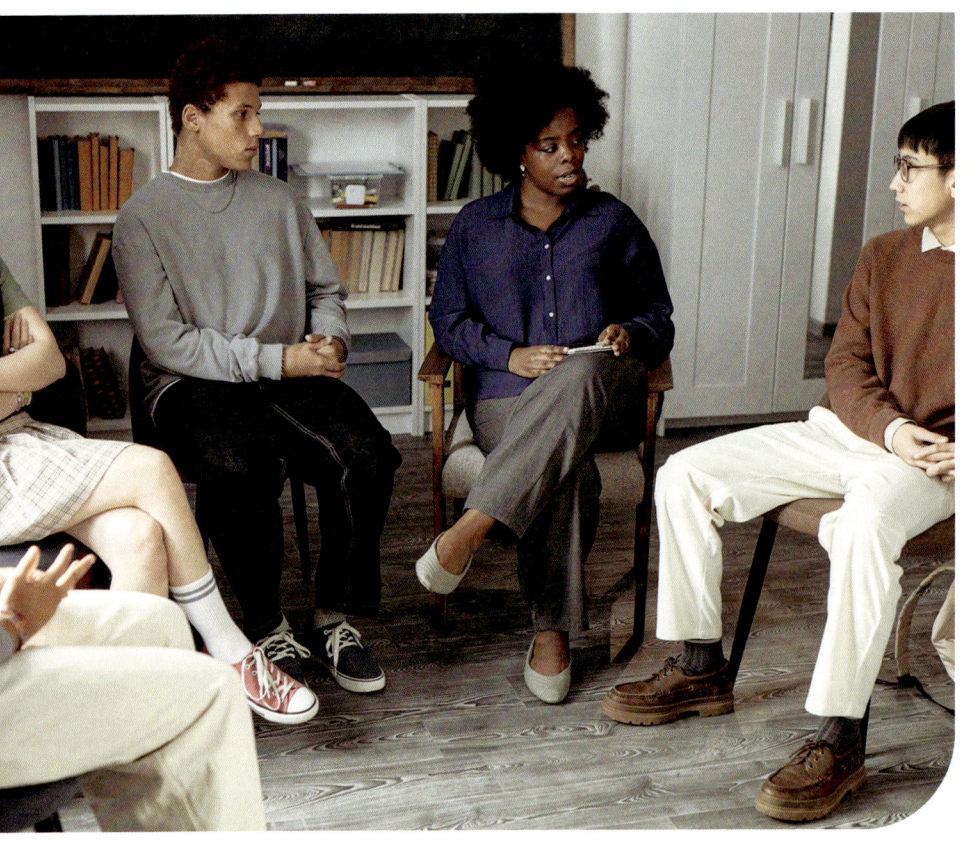

OTHER KINDS OF SUPPORT

Strategies in addition to treatment may help teens cope with SAD. Support groups are one option. A support group is a meeting of people who share an issue in common. Support groups for SAD bring people with the condition together. Members of the group can talk about their experiences with SAD. Listening to other people's thoughts and feelings can help a person understand their own.

    A teen's therapist may be able to connect them with a local support group. Teens may also be able to search for support groups on the internet. Some groups are held online. The Anxiety & Depression Association of America (ADAA) is an organization of mental health professionals. Its website offers a free online support community. Users can discuss their experiences with SAD and related conditions.

    Parents and caregivers of teens with SAD may be able to help them deal with the condition. One way they can help is by not accommodating their teens' fears. Accommodation, in this case, is when a caregiver helps a person in their care avoid what they fear. It is natural for caregivers to want to protect their teens from fear. But accommodation can convince teens that they cannot handle what they fear. This can stand in the way of teens' progress in overcoming their fears.

    Accommodation can come in many forms. A parent of a teen with SAD may

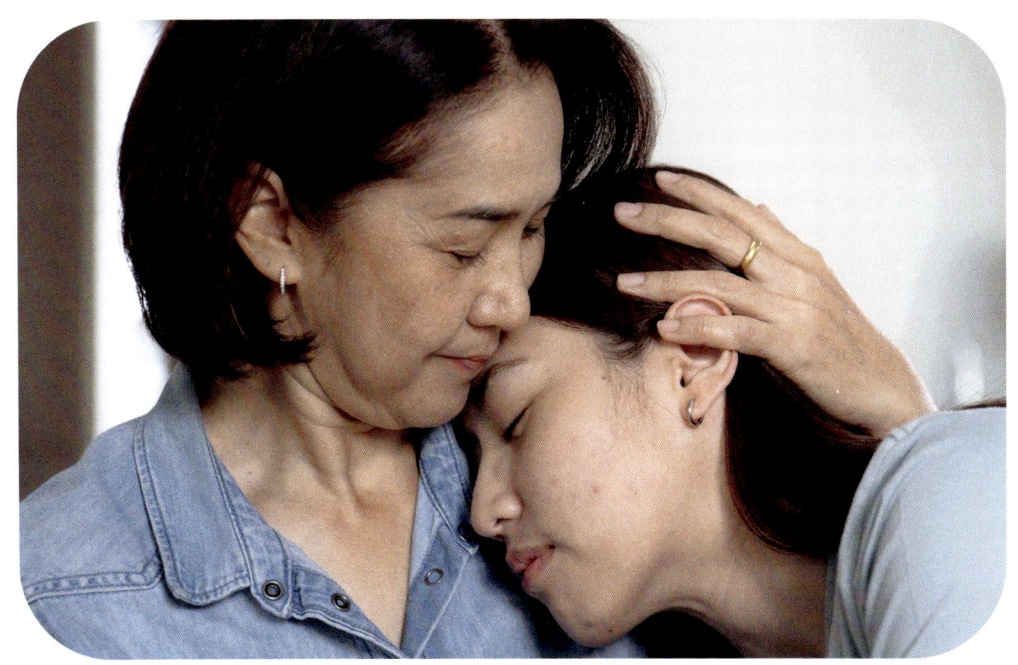

In place of accommodation, caregivers of teens with SAD might listen to their teens' worries and encourage them to feel confident.

order food for them at a restaurant. Or a caregiver may allow a teen to stay home from school. Professionals encourage caregivers to think of the ways they accommodate fears. Then, with teens' permission, the caregivers can work on reducing their accommodation over time.

Teens with SAD who improve their health in other ways may find improvement in

SAD symptoms as well. One study showed that exercise can reduce SAD symptoms when combined with group CBT. Getting enough sleep can also help teens with SAD. Not sleeping well may make people with SAD more likely to avoid social situations.

For teens with SAD, there is hope that things can get better.

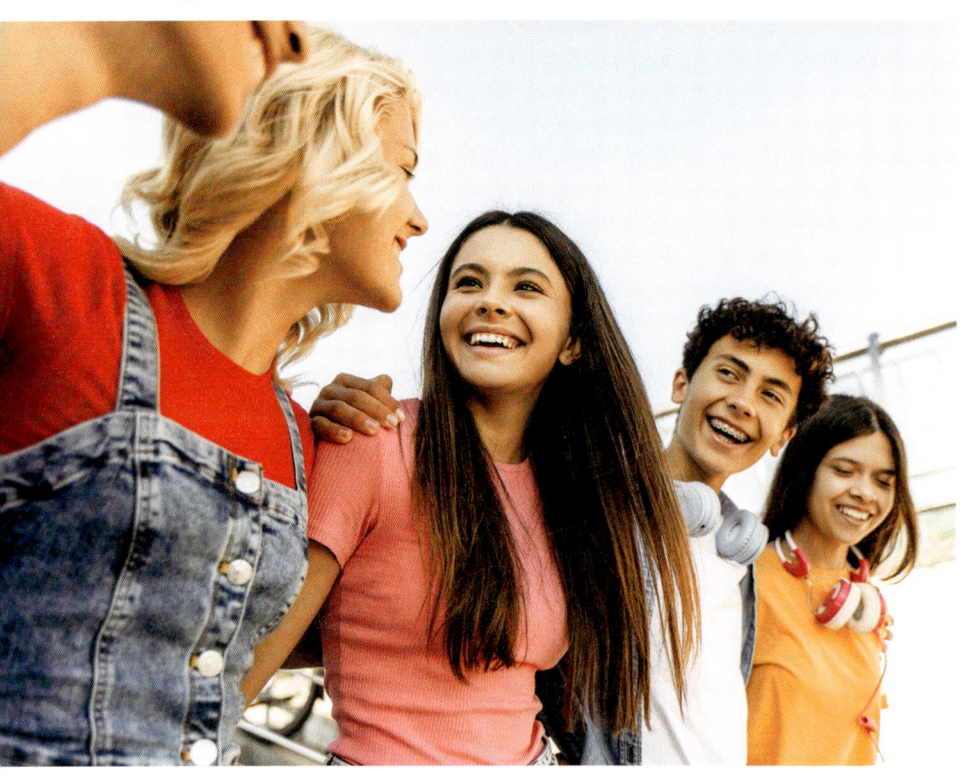

SAD can have many negative effects for teens. It can prevent them from making friends and joining clubs. It can even cause them to avoid school. These effects can seriously disrupt a teen's life.

Treatment can help teens with SAD overcome these effects. Therapy and medication are effective treatments for many teens. Support groups and other strategies may also help. Health care can help a teen with SAD take control of their social life.

GLOSSARY

cognitive
relating to thinking and learning

diagnosed
identified as the cause of symptoms by a medical professional

isolation
the state of being separated from other people

psychiatrists
doctors who treat mental health issues

psychologist
a professional who studies how people think, feel, and behave

ruminate
to think repetitively about negative or troubling feelings

symptoms
signs of a medical condition

trajectory
a path a person or object follows

SOURCE NOTES

INTRODUCTION: GRIDIRON STAR GRAPPLES WITH SOCIAL ANXIETY

1. Quoted in Monique Judge, "Ricky Williams Is Advocating for Mental Health in 'Soul Training,'" *Andscape*, June 16, 2023. https://andscape.com.

CHAPTER ONE: WHAT IS SOCIAL ANXIETY?

2. Quoted in Olivia Guy-Evans, "How Social Anxiety Affects Teens: Signs & How To Help," *SimplyPsychology*, September 19, 2023. www.simplypsychology.org.

CHAPTER TWO: EFFECTS OF SOCIAL ANXIETY

3. Quoted in Guy-Evans, "How Social Anxiety Affects Teens: Signs & How to Help."

4. Mehek Azra, "What's It Like to Be a Teen with Social Anxiety," *Skipping Stones*, March 23, 2021. www.skippingstones.org.

5. Quoted in Laura Bijnsdorp, "Fourteen and Diagnosed with Extreme Social Anxiety," *Growing Up Safe*, September 2023. https://growingupsafe-sxm.com.

6. "'I'm Still Me' — Hilary's Story," *Rethink Mental Illness*, April 22, 2024. www.rethink.org.

CHAPTER THREE: FINDING SUPPORT FOR SOCIAL ANXIETY

7. Quoted in Tori DeAngelis, "Anxiety Among Kids Is on the Rise. Wider Access to CBT May Provide Needed Solutions," *American Psychological Association*, October 1, 2022. www.apa.org.

8. Quoted in Kristen Rogers, "After Years of Debilitating Social Anxiety, a Special Tool Changed My Life," *CNN Health*, April 1, 2022. www.cnn.com.

FOR FURTHER RESEARCH

BOOKS

Mary Bates, *Teen Guide: Depression*. BrightPoint Press, 2026.

Where to Start: A Survival Guide to Anxiety, Depression, and Other Mental Health Challenges. Rocky Pond Books, 2023.

Philip Wolny, *Teens Dealing with Mental Illness*. BrightPoint Press, 2025.

INTERNET SOURCES

"A Guide to Social Anxiety Disorder in Teens," *The Horsham Clinic*, January 6, 2025. https://horshamclinic.com.

Shantel Sullivan, "Social Anxiety in Adolescents: 10 Strategies for Building Confidence," *Bright Path*, October 28, 2024. www.brightpathbh.com.

"Teen Mental Health," *MedlinePlus*, July 30, 2024. https://medlineplus.gov.

WEBSITES

Anxiety & Depression Association of America
https://adaa.org

The Anxiety & Depression Association of America (ADAA) is an organization of mental health care professionals dedicated to treating anxiety and depression disorders. Its website contains information and resources for people looking to learn more about these mental health conditions.

Association for Behavioral and Cognitive Therapies
www.abct.org

The Association for Behavioral and Cognitive Therapies brings together mental health care professionals who study and treat psychological conditions. Its website has information for people who want to learn more about psychological conditions. The website also helps connect patients with local professionals.

MedlinePlus
https://medlineplus.gov

MedlinePlus is an official website of the US government. The MedlinePlus website provides information on many mental health topics, including social anxiety disorder.

INDEX

accommodation, 54–56
amygdala, 23
attachment styles, 23–24

biological causes of social anxiety, 20–23
bullying, 25

celebrities with social anxiety, 6–10, 33
cognitive behavioral therapy (CBT), 43–46, 48, 50, 57

depression, 35
diagnosing social anxiety, 9, 15

embarrassment, 18–19, 50
exposure therapy, 46–49

genetics, 20–22

isolation, 10, 12, 20, 26–28, 38, 48

job interviews, 31

panic attacks, 16–18
parenting methods, 23–25
physical symptoms, 16–18

rumination, 19–20

school, 10, 14, 16, 18, 26–32, 42, 47, 55, 57
selective serotonin reuptake inhibitors (SSRIs), 50–53
self-esteem, 32, 38, 48
side effects of SSRIs, 52–53
social skills training (SST), 49
suicide, 36–39
support groups, 40, 53–54, 57

therapy, 9–10, 36, 40, 43–51, 53, 57
twin studies, 21–22

unsafe substance use, 35–36

Williams, Ricky, 6–10

IMAGE CREDITS

Cover: © fizkes/Shutterstock Images
5: © Motortion Films/Shutterstock Images
7: © Kathy Hutchins/Shutterstock Images
8: © insta_photos/Shutterstock Images
11: © AYO Production/Shutterstock Images
13: © SpeedKingz/Shutterstock Images
14: © Pheelings Media/Shutterstock Images
17: © Antonio Guillem/Shutterstock Images
18: © Krakenimages.com/Shutterstock Images
21: © Jes2u.photo/Shutterstock Images
22: © New Africa/Shutterstock Images
25: © PeopleImages.com-Yuri A./Shutterstock Images
27: © Daniel Hoz/Shutterstock Images
29: © Nature's Charm/Shutterstock Images
30: © Stokkete/Shutterstock Images
33 (top): © Leonard Zhukovsky/Shutterstock Images
33 (mid): © DFree/Shutterstock Images
33 (bottom): © Tinseltown/Shutterstock Images
34: © DimaBerlin/Shutterstock Images
35: © New Africa/Shutterstock Images
36: © VH-Studio/Shutterstock Images
37: © Egoitz Bengoetxea/Shutterstock Images
41: © LightField Studios/Shutterstock Images
42: © VH-Studio/Shutterstock Images
45: © New Africa/Shutterstock Images
47: © Monkey Business Images/Shutterstock Images
48: © La Famiglia/Shutterstock Images
51: © Sonis Photography/Shutterstock Images
52: © SeventyFour/Shutterstock Images
55: © Chay_Tee/Shutterstock Images
56: © AYO Production/Shutterstock Images

ABOUT THE AUTHOR

Mary Gerard lives in St. Paul, Minnesota. Gerard loves cheering on the local Twin Cities teams and the Wisconsin Badgers. She also enjoys binging streaming shows, traveling, playing with her puppy, and watching her kids play sports.